I0440861

Ecstasy Unshackled: Great Lovemaking Made Simple

By Ven Marsman

Createspace Edition

Table of Contents

Dedication

This educational book is dedicated to couples who genuinely care for each other deeply; and committed to make their relationships exciting and long-lasting. This could benefit especially those who may be experiencing some challenges with physical intimacy—and needing an effective catalyst for renewed vigor in their relationships each and every day.

Foreword

The definition of "great lover" is debatable and could be different for different people. The same is true for the meaning of "making love" and "having sex". The politically-correct explanation may be that everyone is entitled to her or his personal opinion. With due respect, while the book can be useful to any responsible adult couples, the essence of this book originates from the author's perspective as a married man.

For the purpose of this book, having sex is defined simply as the physical act of sexual intercourse to satisfy sexual urge or need---with or without emotional attachment. Making love, on the other hand, is more holistic. It is defined as a complete package of passionate actions by a man with an unselfish desire to fully satisfy a woman by giving her his undivided and unhurried attention; and gifting her with extremely pleasurable intimate emotional and physical experience---including an ecstatic conclusion from sexual union—setting aside his needs as secondary. By being unselfish, he becomes a confident and empowered lover! He who attains this high level of lovemaking accomplishment is a great lover!

This condensed but very informative book is intended to benefit you, married couples. It doesn't matter whether you are madly in love with each other, just going through the motions, or somewhere in between. Perhaps you married when you were too young or too old. It doesn't really matter! It doesn't even matter whether you have money or not! This is a great social equalizer...because it works equally well whether you are super rich or extremely poor! The information contained in this book could, in dramatic ways, potentially improve, revive or even revolutionize the intimacy of your physical relationships.

Marriage can be complicated. Everybody knows that it requires commitment and maturity, yet a lot of people have a hard time living up to their vows. There's a lot of moving parts that can go wrong, and if the couple are not persistent and genuinely committed to stick with each other for the long haul—divorce may just be a matter of time.

Post-marriage experience can be challenging. It was reported that in the U.S., 50% of first marriages, 67% of second, and 74% of third marriages end in divorce (Forest Institute of

Professional Psychology in Springfield, Missouri as cited in the link www.divorcerate.org; accessed 12/07/2012). It is really sad that this situation is becoming like an epidemic!

Reasons for divorce abound. Some are irreconcilable differences, incompatibilities, physical intimacy problems, infidelity, financial problems, and so on and so forth. Problems on physical intimacy are often listed as one of the top 5 reasons for divorce. This highlights the importance of a healthy and satisfying sexual relationship between married couples. It is disheartening to note that deteriorating physical relationships and unfulfilled sexual needs break marriages, when in most cases something can be done to minimize, if not prevent them. This idea is the central driving force behind the writing of this book.

This book is intended for two groups of married people: first, for couples who already have healthy physical relationship but would like to take their intimacy to the next level; and second, for couples who may have challenges on physical intimacy but would like to give it a second chance! Both couples could benefit greatly from this book.

While the situation may be different from one couple to another, the author hopes that mastering the great-lover-technique presented in this book will serve as catalyst for physical intimacy that strengthen the marital bond of couples, thereby increasing their chances of long-term success.

With that, the author would have accomplished his original goal in writing this book.

CHAPTER 1
The Ven Marsman Maneuver (VMM)

Congratulations!

You are now ready to turn the key to becoming a great lover! First things first, please don't forget to consult your doctor to make sure you are healthy enough to withstand the rigors of high-intensity great lovemaking. You need to see your doctor, too, if you have erectile dysfunction (ED).

This book presents the unique great-lover-technique, which I call Ven Marsman Maneuver or "VMM" for short. VMM transcends the traditional idea of sex...as it includes a specific set of steps that captures the true essence of great lovemaking.

VMM offers the following potential benefits:

• It guarantees longer and more exciting lovemaking;

• It allows better control of the tempo of lovemaking;

• It prevents pre-mature ejaculation;

- Your size doesn't really matter!
- It increases her chances of having great orgasm/s every time you make love;
- It improves chances of simultaneous orgasms;
- It enables her to have a highly pleasurable intimate physical experience;
- It makes her fully-satisfied---physically and emotionally;
- It makes her very proud of you;
- It boosts your manly confidence; and
- It makes you really proud of yourself!

To sum it all, VMM could make your love life more dynamic and exceptionally exciting! I would venture to say that this may be the single most important discovery that could make a revolutionary improvement in your love life, bar none.

This could be the beginning of an enriched and fulfilling physical relationship with her! I encourage you to go for it! You have everything to gain! I know, because I have been there. My wife and I have been happily married for over 10 years before I discovered and developed VMM. Only then have we started to really experience the ultimate enjoyment of physical intimacy.

VMM could empower couples to be in a honeymoon- mood every day! I simply could not think of any better alternative! And I bet you would feel the same way once you experienced it! And now, it is your turn to become a great lover! If I can do it, I know you can do it!

Let us begin....

The great-lover-technique, called VMM, consists of a unique set of steps for great lovemaking that I discovered and developed personally through the years. It combines the following two basic and essential components:

ONE: MAN'S ABILITY TO INCREASINGLY BUILD-UP THE WOMAN'S DESIRE AND ANTICIPATION FOR PENETRATION; AND MAN'S DISCIPLINED SELF-CONTROL AND PATIENCE IN

TEMPORARY HOLDING OFF THE ACTUAL
PENETRATION; AND

TWO: TIMELY AND CONTROLLED
CONTRACTION OF THE MAN'S PUBOCOCCYGEAL
MUSCLE, THE MUSCLE RESPONSIBLE FOR
CONTROLLING URINATION.

This book revolves around these two
deceptively simple techniques! The secret lies in
the unique technique of implementation. It is very
important that components one and two be
combined in order to experience the genuine
ecstasy possible from VMM lovemaking technique.
Item one is the key component and item two is the
'icing on the cake' that will add intensity to the
whole ecstatic experience.

If you are interested, you can find more
information and a more detailed description of the
pubococcygeal muscle (also called PC muscle)
under the link:

http://en.wikipedia.org/wiki/Pubococcygeus_musc le (accessed 12/07/2012). Throughout the text below, I will call this special muscle the great-lover-muscle, to emphasize its function under VMM.

The main objective of this book is to share with you the tested and proven step-by-step VMM, a great lovemaking technique that I found truly effective in making full use of this great-lover-muscle to your advantage and to her extreme delight every time you make love!

"Kegel" exercises---named after Dr. Arnold Kegel, is the typical way to strengthen the great-lover-muscle. While you will only need the simplified exercises included in this book for the VMM, in case you are interested in more comprehensive and possibly more scientific details you can see the reference at the link: http://en.wikipedia.org/wiki/Kegel_exercise (accessed 12/07/2012). This exercise is applicable to both men and women. The exercise has various health advantages, but in this book I will focus specifically on its function in VMM. The rest is beyond the scope of this book. Now, let's look at how you can develop the VMM skill...that is, in case you don't have it yet.

CHAPTER 2
Simplified Exercise for the Great-Lover-Muscle

This daily exercise for beginners is designed to develop personal control on the muscle. Please note that this can be modified to tailor-fit your personal needs and wants.

Practice contracting your great-lover-muscle, as if you were holding back the flow of your urine.

This step is very simple; and at first, you may think it is too easy! But I can assure you that this serves a very important purpose! You need to be patient. Practice makes perfect. Repetition works wonders. You can do this step every morning and every evening, or whenever you have the time during the day. This is a very small price to pay for you to reach your goal of becoming a great lover! Would you agree?

• For days 1-2: Take a deep breath, and do 5 contractions of your great-lover-muscle at a time.

Repeat this step for 2 minutes—resting and deep breathing for a couple of seconds in between.

- For days 3-4: Do 10 contractions of your great-lover-muscle at a time. Repeat this step for 3 minutes. Don't forget to breathe!

- For days 5-7: Do 15 contractions of your great-lover-muscle at a time. Repeat this step for 4 minutes. Maintain breathing at regular intervals!

- For best results: repeat the last step for another week. After that, you can do the exercise at your convenience---practically anytime, anywhere! By this time, the exercise should have been natural to you; and can be part of your daily routine. And nobody will even notice!

In fact, if you are up to the task, you can do the same exercise when you actually urinate. Try to temporarily hold the flow of your actual urine at convenient intervals by flexing your great-lover-muscle. See how good you are!

The more you do it, the better control you will develop over your great-lover-muscle! That should be your ultimate objective. Note that this exercise can be incorporated with any exercise regimen you already have---without too much extra effort. If you are already doing cardio and other stamina-building exercises---that would be fantastic! You are definitely much better off than most of the average guys!

In case you already know how to control the flexing of your great-lover-muscle right off the bat---that would be great! You may not even have the need for the contraction exercises described above! You can proceed directly to the implementation of the VMM in Chapter 3—which is the most exciting part!

CHAPTER 3
Actual Application of the 16-Step Unique VMM!

Now, it's time for you to get her involved. I can assure you that this will be a big surprise for her! By this time, I presume she has no idea yet of what you are into. But she will know for sure---sooner than later! Guaranteed! Right now, you just need to concentrate on controlling the contraction of your great-lover-muscle.

You will try your best to focus on satisfying her to the fullest...and giving her an extreme sexual pleasure that she may not have experienced in her life! In so doing, you will, for sure, feel a great sense of   accomplishment--and achieve great sexual pleasure, too! Let her be the judge of your performance in bed! Based on personal experience, I bet she will detect the big difference—to the point that she can no longer help but ask you about it!

I cannot stress it enough that you need to focus on her! Feel, look, and listen! "Read" her body language at all times. This will tell you whether or not you are doing the right moves the right way at the right time!

And now, without much further ado, here are the steps for the real thing!

STEP ONE.

Perform foreplay for 10 to 15 minutes or longer, as much as possible. I'm sure you already know that this is an essential part of great lovemaking; and is very important especially for women. This phase will get her more sensitive and accommodating to your next moves.

You need to multi-task. Use your lips, your tongue, your palm, your fingers, your arms, and your legs to explore her entire body. Very important: Be passionate and gentle!

You can concentrate on the most erogenous parts of her body such as her inner thighs, areas around her vagina (but not the clitoris, just yet), her nipples, the lower and side parts of her breasts, her back, her neck, her ears, and her hair. Take your time. Caress the rest of her body--from head to toe. Express genuine appreciation as often as you can. Find something about her to compliment---her hair...her amazing smell...her soft lips...her smooth skin... etc.! I know some men may be uncomfortable doing this; and may prefer to just keep quiet and just do the moves. That is fine, too—but they miss potential benefits.

One benefit is that she will be more relaxed. Another good thing is that she will feel great because this action shows that you are attracted to her; and totally focused on her! This also indicates that you appreciate and respect her; and that you are interested in satisfying her, first and foremost, instead of yourself. This makes you a great-lover-in-the-making!

Under normal condition, the longer the foreplay is, the longer and the better the lovemaking is. This is also one subtle way to save your energy and prevent pre-mature ejaculation which is a typical problem in some men. This gives you a better control of the tempo of the lovemaking session.

Through all of the next steps, it is very important that you caress her body constantly. Continuous motion and sustained touching is a must! Again, you need to read her body language at all times, so you can adjust and use moves that best works with her.

STEP TWO.

Determine her level of arousal by slowly and gently sliding your hand from the knee level upwards to her inner thigh and along the side of her vagina, with your middle finger pressing slightly inside her---to feel her wetness. By this time, most likely you would already have an erection.

Once she is already juiced up and ready---tickle her clitoris with the tip of the head---repeat, just the tip of the head---of your erect penis by slowly and steadily sliding it back and forth for one minute or longer. She is most sensitive down there!

You can do this important penis tip-teasing move faster and slower alternately—depending on what her body language dictates. If you are getting tired after doing step for some time, you can save some energy by holding your penis with one hand and use this hand to slide your penis tip back and forth slowly, rather than move your entire body for this step.

STEP THREE.

At this point, her body language may tell you that she wants penetration. But make sure you hold off! Be patient! Don't penetrate yet! Just continue, using your lips and tongue, to explore sensitive parts of her body while you are doing step 2.

Bear in mind: It's all about building up her anticipation and desire for penetration; and you holding off temporarily! Maintain your disciplined self-control! That is the key, my friend! Bear with me, but I probably need to repeat that reminder many times for it to sink in!

STEP FOUR.

Slowly stick the head, repeat--just the head--of your penis, in her vagina. Thrust the head in and out for one minute or more. By this time, she might have been literally begging you for full penetration! But make sure you do not yield to her, at least not yet! Be patient! Again, this penis head-teasing move is crucially important!

It should come as no surprise if she tries penetration herself by arching her hips towards you! But bear in mind, I repeat, that you need to resist and avoid penetration---albeit in a subtle way.

Just continue teasing her vagina with the head of your penis--and using your lips, tongue, and hands to caress other erogenous parts of her body. She may be totally aroused and frantic at this point...but again, just hold off! Be patient! Control your urge to give in to her wishes! At least, not yet!

I Repeat...Be patient, my friend! I cannot stress it enough! You are increasingly building up her anticipation and desire for your full penetration moves! That is the main purpose of holding off!

I know I'm being absurdly repetitious! But if that's what it takes to get you to learn this stuff and make it part of your inner self...I don't care! I don't want you to fail her! You owe it to her! I need you to get it done! And lastly, I don't want you to fail me as a teacher!

Steps 1 through 4 will ensure that she will be extremely sensitive to, and in great anticipation of, and very accommodating of, your next moves!...your great-lover moves!

STEP FIVE.

Now, choose any lovemaking position that you both are comfortable with. Initially, I would suggest the missionary position (where she lies on her back with her legs apart while you lower yourself on top of her supporting your weight with your elbows), as it will give you better control of the pace of the Ven Marsman Maneuver (VMM).

Later on, you will find out that the typical woman-astride position (where you lie on your back and she sits on you) is also an excellent choice for this step.

Another good position, especially if you are already tired, is the spoon, where both of you lie on your sides facing the same direction, with you penetrating her from behind, allowing full body contact--with your hands free to caress her breasts, her face, her neck and her hair.

In fact, you can apply the next steps to practically any position you are familiar and comfortable with. Discussion of other lovemaking positions is beyond the scope of this book because I presume you already know some of the basic positions. At any rate, you can always learn more on your own at your convenience!

STEP SIX.

Now, in one slow stroke, stick the entire length of your penis into her vagina; stop at full penetration position; press firmly; don't move!

This simple action will be extremely delightful for her, considering her prolonged wait and anticipation for penetration! It is not uncommon for her to let go off a big sigh of relief at this point! She has no idea that this is only the beginning of an unforgettable ecstatic ending!

STEP SEVEN.

Now is the time to apply the contraction exercise you have been doing every day with your great-lover-muscle! This is a must step in the VMM! While still at full penetration position and pressing firmly (step 6), contract your great-lover-muscle a few times at one-second intervals! Watch her amazing reactions! Remember, she would have been very sensitive at this point after going through steps 1-6.

Continue the contraction for 30 seconds or more. Meanwhile, don't forget to use your lips, tongue, and hands to caress other accessible parts of her body for extra sensation. I can assure you that she would have been absolutely frantic at this point---almost begging for you to give it all to her! And that's when you know you are doing great, so far, my friend!

STEP EIGHT.

Now, withdraw your penis slowly, up until the tip is just touching her vagina slightly. Slowly stick your penis again, but this time only halfway in. Thrust it in and out steadily...halfway only...10 times or more!

STEP NINE.

Then penetrate fully; and repeat step 7. At this point she would have been extremely frantic and ecstatic—and could be begging you for more! That is great! And totally expected! Tap your shoulders because that means you are doing really great! Congratulations for getting this far, my friend!

NOW, FOR ANY OF THE FOLLOWING STEPS, YOU HAVE THE OPTION TO REACH CLIMAX (ORGASM)! YOU NEED TO BE PREPARED FOR A HIGHLY-EXPLOSIVE CLIMAX---HERS AT FIRST, AND THEN POSSIBLY YOURS!

Note: If privacy is important to you, make sure that you make love in a completely sound-proof location because it is highly likely that you may not be able to stop her from making loud sounds and moans! Otherwise, go for it! It is entirely up to you!

STEP TEN.

Now comes the right time to give it all to her! Thrust the entire length of your penis in and out of her vagina's depth---in slow strokes. Contract your great-lover-muscle during your inward stroke! This will give her an extremely delightful sensation!

It is not uncommon for her to arch her hips towards you, wanting to follow your slow outward stroke to maintain contact with your penis. That should give you more confidence that you are doing it right! You can do this step for one minute or more; and you can choose to extend this step until both of you reach orgasm! Again, it's up to you.

For your possible interest, let me explain the uniqueness of contracting your great-lover-muscle. What happens during this stroke is a combination of two penile movements: First, the ordinary vertical and downward sliding movement of your penis along the sensitive walls of her vagina; and second, the special horizontal and spasmodic movement of your penis--due to girth enlargement and tip movement, as you contract your great-lover-muscle.

Combined, these two movements will give her a special ecstatic feeling---one that, I bet, she has never experienced in her whole life! Before proceeding any further, let me point out something that may not be too obvious. Practically all of us men know when we reach climax, as it is a very pleasurable sensation and is usually accompanied by ejaculation of semen. But how do you know when she is about to reach orgasm? That's a very good question!

The signs may vary from woman to woman, but some of the possibilities are listed below:

• You will feel her uncontrolled, almost violent, hip thrusts; • She will show heavy breathing, and moans;

• If you slow down, she will likely say "please don't stop!";

• Her eyes may open wider;

• Or she may simply say, "I'm coming!"

• Once she reaches climax, she may close her eyes; and her body may become limp.

• When you try to continue thrusting in and out after climax, she may say "please stop!" because by this time her vagina will have been super sensitive to touch!

• Also during climax, a woman can:
- feel a spasmodic clitoral sensation;
- be light-headed;
- have blurry vision;

- have a feeling of tingles throughout her body; and
- experience lightness of body

Now, let's resume the VMM step...

STEP ELEVEN.

If you choose not to climax in step 10, and you are already tired, you can stop the penis thrusting in-and-out strokes temporarily, and simply go back to step 7.

STEP TWELVE.

Otherwise, continue and do a modified in-and-out penis thrusting movement---slow in and slow out strokes at first, followed by slow in and quick/snappy out strokes. Do this about 10 times or more. I bet she will beg for you not to stop! And it will be an amazing feeling for you!

STEP THIRTEEN.

To heighten her delight, move sideways back and forth while you are doing the in-and-out stroke. To make her feel your "bigness" and "hardness" even more, encourage her (in a subtle way) to put her legs closer together while you assume a modified missionary/man-astride position with your legs lying outside of, and "pinning", both her legs—while you support the weight of your upper body with your elbows set below her armpits.

Continue the in-and-out thrusting of penis, with contraction of your great-lover-muscle during the inward stroke. This step is especially helpful if she already lacks the youthful vaginal "tightness" due to childbirth, among other reasons.

She will be pleasantly surprised because she will feel like a "virgin" again! You can do this for a minute or more. Again, you can choose to continue doing this step until both of you reach climax!

STEP FOURTEEN.

If you are shorter that her, and the height difference allows it, you may use a unique and special maneuver. Try to arch your body and support your weight with your pointed elbows resting beside her, slightly below her breast level---with your hands free and resting lightly on her breasts.

Now, you can kiss her lips and simultaneously massage her nipples with the tip of your thumb and index fingers and her breasts gently with your palm and fingers---while you are in penetration mode! Believe me...this simultaneous three-pronged maneuver is superbly unique in every way! In fact, if you are much shorter than her, you can even use your tongue to play with and/or suck her nipples gently while you are in penetration mode; and you can simultaneously massage her breasts, and her other sensitive parts like her face, her neck, her ears, her hair, etc.!

Can you imagine the amazing sensation those simultaneous moves would give her! And the pleasure it would give you! I can assure you that the simultaneous effects of these three moves combined will give her extra special sensation that only this unique maneuver can accomplish! That would be ecstasy beyond belief!

Knowing this unique possibility, I bet this is probably the only time that you wish you were a lot shorter than she is! Sorry for you, tall guys! You have no chance to do this maneuver with your equally tall or shorter ladies—without dangerously straining your neck! I say, don't even try to do it!

This is counter-intuitive because traditionally, most women prefer taller men. And shorter men generally feel inadequate and inferior! I would venture to guess that I maybe the very first one to come up with this revolutionary idea---that only a man relatively shorter than the woman can possibly give that woman this uniquely amazing ecstatic experience!

So from now on---you, short and shorter guys have something to rejoice about! Learn and practice this unique triple maneuver! When you become good at this, you will realize that, yes, height really matters...only that---now, it is in your favor! How is that for a change!

OK, so much for that diversion. Let's resume...

STEP FIFTEEN.

To conserve your energy, an option would be for you to encourage her to do the typical woman-astride position while you are simply lying on your back—allowing her to have full control of the pace and depth of penetration. Here, she does the penetration herself by sitting up straight on top of you--facing you. She basically does the in-and-out thrusting as she pleases, at her own tempo. Now you are relatively relaxed and comfortable, and have the perfect opportunity to fully concentrate on contracting your great-lover-muscle! Contract your great-lover-muscle during her inward stroke. Focus all your energy—concentrate! Do it all for her!

Some women like to assume this position because it gives them a sense of dominance and control over us men, giving them more intensity during great lovemaking. This position also increases the chance of your penis "touching" her illusive G-spot---if that is important to you. Although not commonly understood by many, touching that spot is supposed to give her extra sensation. You be the judge.

Another big benefit of this position, of course, is that your two hands are free to titillate her nipples, or you can kiss and suck them gently if you can reach them, and caress other parts of her body. That would be very sensually enjoyable!

Meanwhile, continue to contract your great-lover-muscle during the inward stroke—as she continues the in-and-out thrusts. Again, you can continue to do this step until both of you reach orgasm!

Note: If simultaneous orgasm is important to you, you will increase your chances of achieving it if the two of you coordinate by giving each other clear signals when you are about "to come"—and then focus all your energy to maintain consistent movements, building up "tension" and excitement until you reach orgasm!

On the other hand, if you feel like you are about "to come" too soon (ejaculate pre-maturely) in any given position or movement, you can hold it off by doing either or a combination of two things: first, by slowing down your tempo; and/or second, by changing positions smoothly. This will temporarily cool down the tension and prolong your lovemaking session. Make sure you do this without being too obvious—maintaining your "connection" with her by switching to foreplay moves gradually. You can do this on-and-off maneuver as long as you want, and as long as she would tolerate it, based on her body language!

And then once you are ready, be prepared for the most explosive climax she will ever have! Just a reminder: Most likely, she will have her orgasm/s first in many occasions if you strictly follow the VMM steps. It is crucial for you to be aware that her vagina is extremely sensitive immediately after climax—and you need to be very careful when you decide to reach your own orgasm after hers.

Again, read her body language and "check" whether you think she can still withstand continued in-and-out penis moves—or if she needs more time to rest before resuming your lovemaking session. However, based on experience, chances are that she would encourage you to have your own climax regardless of how sensitive she feels. Satisfying you is important to her, too. And who knows, she may even have a second orgasm herself!

STEP SIXTEEN.

Lastly, post-play after climax is very important, too. Make sure you don't go to sleep, nor leave her right away, after you "come"! Continue to be passionate and tender with her. Hug her and make her feel your protective warmth. Make her feel secure in your arms. Make her feel appreciated in your own special way. Be mindful that her body may be sensitive to touch. Again, read her body language. I certainly hope that you should be very good at doing that already at this point.

It is quite important for her to know that you are very pleased, fulfilled, and satisfied as she is. Depending on your personalities, sweet nothings may not be too bad at this point!

CONGRATULATIONS! YOU DID IT!

Are you now a believer that the Ven Marsman Maneuver (VMM) works? I'm sure you are! IT REALLY DOES! AND IN A BIG WAY!

CHAPTER 4
An Afterthought

After the two of you have rested from that great lovemaking experience, made possible by VMM, chances are that she will wonder how in the world you are able to do that! Of course, you may choose not to reveal how you developed your "secret" new-found skill--leaving her wondering how your transformation happened!

Either way, I bet she will feel totally satisfied and fulfilled! The advantage of telling her about the VMM is that, at some point, you may even be able to encourage her to do the same exercises that you have done.

That is, for her to also strengthen and develop control over her own great-lover-muscle...that she can later use the same way as you do during your future great lovemaking sessions! And believe me---that would really be doubly special treat for both of you! Those timely simultaneous contractions of two sets of touching great-lover-muscles could create an unbelievably explosive great lovemaking experience that is hard to put into words!

Presented in this book are the fundamental steps of the great-lover's technique called Ven Marsman Maneuver (VMM). Bear in mind that this technique is not set on stone. It is flexible. You are free to do reasonable modification or combination of the steps, depending on your preference as a couple. It's your choice. It's entirely up to you!

Don't be afraid to experiment! The possibilities are many! Do what mutually works for both of you! Note that you can also prolong your great lovemaking by doing any or a combination of the following: extended foreplay, holding off climax, and repeating or prolonging VMM steps. At first, you may feel like you are not as good as you would like to be, but like any other endeavors, you will become better through repetition and practice.

During great lovemaking, the key is to be sensitive to her reactions, and be guided by what satisfies her the most. Use moves that give her the most pleasure. By all means, try to give it all to her ...at the right time! In short, focus on giving her what she needs and wants first...and surely you will get what you need and want in turn!

THAT IS THE REAL SECRET OF A GREAT LOVER! BECOME ONE, AND SHE WILL LIKELY STICK WITH YOU THROUGH THICK AND THIN...

Congratulations! You now hold the key to becoming a great lover! Practice it! Be great at it! And enjoy it fully, my friend! CHEERS!

About the Author

The author is a conservative one-woman man! That may not be too exciting for some people in these modern times---but he is committed to remain that way. He has been happily married to a wonderful woman who is a great wife, a great lover, a great friend, and a super mom combined. And they truly trust and love one another!

He is just an ordinary guy who takes pride in honesty and great work ethic at anything he sets his mind to accomplish. He is a straight shooter who says what he thinks, and expresses what he feels freely! He personally learned and perfected the technique presented in this book exclusively with his wife! He strongly believes that if it has worked for them—it will work for any couple!

Interestingly, where he came from, talking about sex was taboo. As a young boy and until he was about twelve years old, he had absolutely no idea about sex! It seemed as though what happened in the bedroom was the privy of adults. Sex was not taught in school, nor discussed at home. He was on his own as far as this topic was concerned. His activities revolved strictly around home, school, and playground! As a result, he was so shy and naïve, you won't believe it! For one, it was unbelievable that he thought kissing caused pregnancy! What an ignorant young boy he was! But you can't really blame the poor guy…the internet was yet to be invented then!

He learned about sex only from readings initially, and later from close friends. Years passed by and he tried to gain knowledge on the subject as much as he can.

Fortunately, by the time he became an adult and got married, he made sure he knew what he was doing---at least on paper! Not surprisingly, it was a case of trial and error at first…until he got it right! Eventually, he actually became pretty good at it! Good for her!

He started writing the first part of this book years ago because he wanted to share with others his amazing journey to developing great marital physical intimacy. He thought that rather than being taboo, this topic should be discussed openly among responsible adults. But for some reason, he set the book project aside; and forgot all about it due to demands of job and other priorities. He also did not have any idea how to have a book published!

Years passed by, and one day while he was shuffling the contents of his old idle briefcase, to his amazement he saw the original draft manuscript! He was so excited to revisit what he originally started to write---and it renewed his personal desire to share it with others. Actually, the delay may have been beneficial because through the years, he has honed up his knowledge and skills on the subject. He believes that he is now uniquely qualified to teach this special subject to others!

What drives him to write this condensed but very informative book is his desire to help married men develop the ability to make their wives experience genuine full intimacy in their physical relationship. In so doing, men will experience great fulfillment, too. He hopes that the unique lovemaking skills learned from this book will be used responsibly, and not encourage rampant promiscuity.

Physical intimacy is not everything, but it is a pre-requisite for a successful and long-lasting married life. Oftentimes, it can impact even the other important non-physical aspects of a couple's life. It is a quest that, the author believes, all serious married couples need to pursue.

All the best!

Ven Marsman

Disclaimer

This book is designed to provide condensed information based on the author's perspective. It is not intended to present all the information that is otherwise available, but instead to complement and supplement other references. Each user is urged to tailor-fit the information to individual needs. Every effort has been made to make this book as accurate as possible. However, this is not designed to be a literary gem, but rather a reference that provides practical, actionable and effective techniques.

There may be mistakes, both typographical and in content— hence this text should be used only as a general guide and not as the ultimate source of information. The sole purpose of this book is to educate. As such, the author shall have neither liability nor responsibility to any person or entity with respect to any loss or damage caused, or alleged to have been caused, directly or indirectly, by the information contained in this book.

www.ingramcontent.com/pod-product-compliance
Lightning Source LLC
Chambersburg PA
CBHW■71359310526
45790CB00019B/1632